Muted Hunger

Understanding Anorexic Thoughts

by
Amber Lewis

Muted Hunger

Understanding Anorexic Thoughts

Contents

Introduction

An exploration into the secretive and tortuous realm of Anorexia Nervosa beckons us on a journey that extends far beyond mere statistics and clinical terms; it demands an understanding of the real and harrowing narrative that unfolds within the minds of those afflicted. This book seeks to illuminate the intricate and often misunderstood thought processes that dominate the lives of individuals struggling with this debilitating disorder, providing a lighthouse of knowledge for parents and support workers as they navigate through the stormy psyche of loved ones fighting an invisible battle. Part scientific inquiry, part motivational guide, the prose you are about to encounter synthesizes deeply researched insights with an unwavering commitment to empowering readers. It is a testament to the resilience of the human spirit and a call to action for informed, compassionate support. With each page, we delve into a realm where courage meets vulnerability, and recovery becomes a tangible horizon.

The Voices of Anorexia: Inside the Anorexic Mind

Embedded deep within the labyrinth of the anorexic mind lies a persistent echo chamber of voices, a chorus that chants with the beat of self-imposed discipline and the urgent whispers of self-denial. At its core, anorexia nervosa is not merely about the physical act of restricting food but about a relentless mental skirmish. This chapter ventures to unravel these tangled threads of thought, to give a voice to those silent conversations that so powerfully influence actions and shape perceptions. The fabric of this disorder is woven with complex patterns of control and an almost paradoxical sense of desperation that those on the outside struggle to comprehend. Delving into the anorexic mind reveals a tumultuous internal dialogue—one where distorted self-command encounters an unending search for self-worth through self-starvation. At its heart, understanding this dialogue is paramount for parents, friends, and support workers eager to step into the flickering shadows of the anorexic psyche, to shine a light on the unseen battles and to empower with empathy and hope.

Understanding the Internal Dialogues

As we delve deeper into the labyrinth of the anorexic mind, it becomes paramount to unpack the complex internal dialogues that play out within individuals suffering from Anorexia Nervosa. These conversations can range from self-castigating critiques to deceptive rationalizations, all of which reinforce the disorder's grip on the mind and behavior of the person. At first glance, these inner voices may seem monolithic, but a closer examination reveals a multifaceted battle for control and identity.

The inner dialogues of someone with anorexia often revolve around themes of worth, success, and the illusion of power. These individuals can't help but incessantly tally calories, view food as the enemy, and see each pound lost as a victory in a twisted game of self-discipline. What might start as a whisper of "I need to be thin" amplifies into deafening declarations of "I must control my body" to exist within the narrow confines of perceived societal ideals or personal standards.

These dialogues aren't merely passive self-talk; they shape behaviors that can have life-threatening consequences. Scientific research suggests that the positive feedback loop created by the anorexic voice and subsequent weight loss acts on the dopamine pathways, reinforcing the disordered behaviors. It is a negotiation fraught with biological, psychological, and sociological implications—all converging to form a narrative that drives the anorexia sufferer further into the depths of the disorder. It's crucial to understand these internal discussions not as rational choices, but as compulsions fueled by distorted thinking.

But there is a glimmer of hope. By identifying and understanding these dialogues, parents and support workers can begin to counteract the powerful anorexic voice. They can develop compassionate strategies to help sufferers challenge and reframe these unhealthy narratives. It's an uphill battle, where empathy and patience must supersede frustration, and where the echo of positive reinforcement must grow louder than the whispers of the disorder. Understanding this mental framing is pivotal, as it provides the cornerstone for the cognitive restructuring efforts that are crucial in recovery.

The realm of anorexia is mired in a complex psychological web that requires meticulous untangling. As we shine a light on these shadowy discourses, we pave the way for meaningful intervention. Each stride toward understanding these internal dialogues propels us toward reclaiming the minds and lives devastated by this pernicious disease.

The Battle Between Control and Desperation

It's a constant war that rages in the minds of those struggling with Anorexia Nervosa. For the person engaged in this battle, life becomes a chessboard, with each meal, calorie, and reflection in the mirror a move that could result in victory or defeat. It's a narrative that unfolds each day, fraught with tension and the perpetual quest for control over an environment that feels increasingly uncontrollable. Yet, within this pursuit lies a paradox, for the perceived control is but an illusion, masking a profound sense of desperation.

The dynamics at play are complex and multifaceted, characterizing an internal struggle that for many is both persistent and relentless. Control is often seen as the primary motivator, with individuals believing that by meticulously managing their food intake and body shape, they can achieve a semblance of order in their otherwise chaotic world. However, underlying this is a sea of desperation, a driving force fueled by a fear of gaining weight, a fear of not being good enough, and a fear of losing that very sense of control they so desperately cling to.

In the throes of anorexia, the mind becomes an echo chamber, amplifying worries and bolstering beliefs that one's worth is inextricably tied to their physique. The body becomes a project to be perfected, a canvas upon which they attempt to paint their worth. With each pound lost and each bone that surfaces, the sense of accomplishment is palpable. Yet, the triumph is transient, as satisfaction dissipates with the next meal, the next weighing session, the next glimpse of their body.

This battle is not merely one of willpower or strength. It's a conflict shaped by a distorted self-perception, where the mirror's reflection is not to be trusted, and the scale becomes the ultimate arbiter of success. For someone entrenched in the war against weight, the line between victory and defeat is razor-thin. A bite too many or a pound too heavy, and the battle is lost, triggering an avalanche of self-loathing and guilt.

As much as it is a fight for control, this is equally a struggle for identity. Deep within the confines of an anorexic mindset, there is a yearning to be seen, to be known for more than just the contours of one's body. Yet, the desperation to maintain a fragile façade of thinness often overshadows the intrinsic desire for genuine self-expression and connection.

Feeling trapped in a cycle of restriction and obsession, individuals suffering from anorexia often find themselves at a crossroads between the comfort of familiar habits and the terrifying prospect of change. The thought of relinquishing control is synonymous with stepping into the unknown – an abyss filled with uncertainties that seem more daunting than the deceptive safety of the disorder.

Yet, it's important to understand that this battle is not fought in isolation. The specter of anorexia not only haunts the individual but also casts a shadow over the lives of loved ones and caretakers. Witnessing someone entrenched in this struggle often evokes feelings of helplessness and desperation, creating a parallel narrative where control is equally coveted and challenged. The support network surrounding the sufferer becomes part of the battleground, weaving their own tactics and strategies to counter the disorder's cunning moves.

While the battle between control and desperation seems insurmountable, recovery is not beyond reach. It's achieved through a methodical, compassionate approach that involves understanding the nuanced driving forces behind anorexia. Professionals and support networks must endeavor to create spaces where the person battling anorexia feels safe to explore and express their fears, doubts, and hopes.

Key to this process is the dismantling of the voracious cycle of control and the imposition of starvation. It requires a delicate balance – providing structure and support without further feeding into the narrative of control. It's about guiding them slowly towards a new paradigm where control is not about restriction, but about the ability to make choices that nourish rather than punish the body and soul.

On the road to recovery, it's crucial for individuals to redefine their relationship with food and their bodies. Reintroducing the concept of eating as an act of self-care rather than self-sabotage can be transformative. Meals should be reframed as opportunities for healing and celebration of the body's strength and resilience.

Part of this battle involves rekindling a sense of hope – a belief that life beyond anorexia is not only possible but can be filled with joy and fulfillment. Stirring this hope can come from rediscovering passions and activities that have been pushed aside for the sake of the disorder, offering a lifeline to those drowning in a sea of desperation. A restored sense of purpose can be a powerful antidote to the lure of anorexia.

Over time, as individuals learn to temper their need for control with kindness towards themselves, they begin to see that their value is not weighed on a scale. Every victory, no matter how small, is a step towards liberation from the disorder. Progress may be slow, and relapse is part of the journey, but the pursuit of recovery is a testament to human resilience and the capacity to rise above the internal tempest of control and desperation.

Ultimately, the battle between control and desperation in anorexia is a poignant reminder of the enduring human spirit. It's a fight that demands patience, understanding, and perseverance from both the individual and their support network. It's a journey that, although marked by struggle, can lead to a newfound sense of strength and self-compassion. This is not just a story of survival, but one of transformation – a testament to the fact that from the depths of despair, a new life can emerge, one where control exists but does not dominate, where food is a friend, not an enemy, and where self-worth is unconditional.

Chapter 2:
The Anatomical and Psychological Underpinnings of Anorexia Nervosa

Diving deeper into the mysterious layers of anorexia nervosa leads us to a complex interplay of brain biology and emotional psychology. The human brain, an organ already enigmatic and powerful, responds to starvation with neural changes that often reinforce the disorder's grip on an individual. Starvation impacts neurotransmitter systems and can alter mood, anxiety levels, and reward processing, leading to a self-perpetuating cycle of anorexic behaviors. On the flip side, the psychological aspect is anchored in emotions of fear, guilt, and shame that fuse together and magnify the condition's impact, manifesting in a relentless pursuit of thinness. Understanding the brain's response to persistent eating restriction unravels part of the complicated puzzle of anorexia, providing clues on how to support individuals in rewiring their thoughts and emotional responses. Clinicians and researchers are making strides in disentangling the intricate web of factors that contribute to anorexia, including the potential genetic predisposition and the role of environmental stressors. It's clear that every step towards understanding is a leap towards empowering those afflicted to fight back and reclaim their health.

How the Brain Responds to Starvation

Understanding the physical manifestation of anorexia nervosa on the brain begins with exploring how the brain responds to starvation. When the body is deprived of necessary nutrients, it triggers a cascade of physiological and psychological responses aimed at survival. Specifically, the brain goes through a series of adaptions characterized by changes in structure and functionality.

Neuroimaging studies have shown that starvation can lead to alterations in the brain's gray matter. This vital tissue, responsible for processing information, seems to be adversely affected when the body is undernourished. Researchers speculate that these changes might underpin some of the cognitive deficits observed in anorexia, such as problems with concentration and judgment.

As the starvation persists, changes in neurological functioning begin to mirror the adaptions seen in those undergoing severe stress—it's as if the brain is constantly signaling an alarm. For individuals grappling with anorexia, this heightened state of neural alertness can exacerbate feelings of anxiety and reinforce obsessive thoughts about food and weight.

The brain's chemistry is not immune to the effects of starvation either. Serotonin, a neurotransmitter that modulates mood, sleep, and appetite, can become dysregulated in individuals with anorexia. Low levels of serotonin are often associated with mood disorders and could be intertwined with the depression and anxiety common in anorexia sufferers.

Beyond mood, the neuroendocrine system—which includes hormonal axes like the hypothalamic-pituitary-adrenal (HPA) axis—becomes altered under starvation conditions. The HPA axis is central to stress response and energy regulation. In anorexia, this system can become hyperactive, potentially contributing to the maintenance of restrictive eating behaviors.

One of the brain's most primal areas, the hypothalamus, also gets caught up in the turmoil of starvation. It's intricately involved in regulating hunger and satiety. Starvation can lead to an imbalance in the signaling molecules leptin and ghrelin, which normally help regulate appetite. A disrupted balance between these hormones may contribute to anorexia's characteristic disregard for hunger cues.

Another critical component to consider is cognition. Starvation impacts cognitive function, as the brain requires a constant supply of glucose to perform optimally. People with anorexia often demonstrate cognitive impairments; this is possibly a direct consequence of prolonged starvation which deprives the brain of its primary fuel.

Interestingly enough, even when individuals with anorexia nervosa begin to reintroduce food, the brain's response is not immediate restoration. Instead, there's often a period where the brain is recalibrating its perception of satiety and hunger signals. These signals have often gone disregarded or were misinterpreted during the peak of disorder.

From the psychological perspective, starvation enhances the focus on food-related stimuli. People with anorexia tend to have an amplified response to food-related cues, and thoughts about food can become intrusive and obsessive. This hyper-awareness can perpetuate the cycle of restriction, as individuals may avoid or control food intake to cope with the distressing stimuli.

The brain's reward system, usually responsible for the pleasurable sensation associated with eating, also works differently in those with anorexia. Contrary to what one might expect, it's not just the avoidance of food that may give a sense of accomplishment but often, the denial of hunger itself becomes rewarding.

Recovery from anorexia is as much a psychological journey as it is physical. The concept of neuroplasticity gives hope, suggesting that the brain has the remarkable capacity to heal and rewire itself significantly with proper nourishment and therapeutic intervention.

Additionally, the refeeding process itself necessitates careful consideration. If done too abruptly, it can lead to a potentially fatal condition known as refeeding syndrome. Gradual reintroduction of nutrients is essential for allowing the brain to safely adapt to increased energy intake.

Familial support is crucial through this process. Loved ones need to understand that recovery involves a substantial rewiring of deeply engrained behaviors and thought patterns, all of which hinge on the brain's ability to adapt to new nutrient levels and interruptions to the starvation cycle.

However, it's vital to maintain optimism. Despite the challenges, many individuals do successfully recover from anorexia nervosa, learning to nourish their bodies and live without the oppression of disordered eating hanging over their every thought. With each day of adequate nutrition and psychological support, their brains make tremendous strides towards healing and adapting to a healthier mode of functioning.

In closing, it's paramount that those who support individuals with anorexia nervosa comprehend the complexities of how the brain responds to starvation. Acknowledging and addressing these complications can make the path to recovery less daunting for all involved. With understanding, persistence, and a nourishing environment, the brain's resilience shines through, paving the way for recovery and rejuvenation.

The Emotional Synergy of Anorexia: Fear, Guilt, and Shame

Anorexia nervosa is not just a physical affliction but an emotional storm that rages within the minds of those it grips. In the complex tapestry of emotions that ensnare a person suffering from anorexia, fear, guilt, and shame form a potent triad, often reinforcing each other in a debilitating loop.

Fear in anorexia is multifaceted, involving the terror of weight gain, loss of control over eating, and perhaps deeply rooted fears tied to self-worth and acceptance. It's not simply the act of eating that is feared, but what the act signifies—a potential spiral into chaos and inadequacy.

Guilt is intricately interwoven with this fear, coming to the forefront as soon as an individual with anorexia considers eating "normally" or deviates from their rigid dietary rules. This guilt is often an internal manifestation of perceived failure, a betrayal of their own standards of self-discipline, and a breach of the very rules that they believe keep them grounded.

Shame, distinct yet dependent on fear and guilt, is the pervasive feeling of humiliation and distress over one's perceived inadequacies. In the case of anorexia, the shame may be tied to body image, self-perception, or the belief that succumbing to hunger is a sign of weakness. This shame can be so profound that it overshadows any sense of accomplishment and erodes an individual's self-esteem.

The interplay of fear, guilt, and shame can drive a person into a relentless pursuit of thinness, which is mistakenly perceived as a panacea for these negative emotions. It's a bargaining chip in an internal barter system—thinness in exchange for peace, control, and self-approval. However, these emotions can further entrench the eating disorder, creating a vicious cycle that can seem nearly impossible to break free from.

Understanding this emotional synergy is crucial for parents and support workers. It's not enough to address the physical manifestations of anorexia; the emotional underpinnings are the scaffolding that maintains the disorder. Compassionate and comprehensive care must target these emotional complexities alongside any nutritional or therapeutic interventions.

Early psychological interventions can help untangle the web of fear, guilt, and shame. Strategies such as cognitive-behavioral therapy (CBT) are targeted to challenge and modify unhealthy thoughts and behaviors. Encouragement to confront these emotions in a safe environment allows individuals to process and understand them, undermining their power.

Building resilience against these negative emotions often involves cultivating emotional intelligence, empathy, and self-compassion. Family therapy can play a critical role in creating a supportive environment that validates the individual's feelings without judgment and provides tools for coping that don't involve self-starvation.

Mindfulness practices such as meditation can also offer invaluable benefits. Mindfulness encourages a non-judgmental awareness of the present moment, which in turn can help an individual recognize the ephemeral nature of their thoughts and emotions, including fear, guilt, and shame.

Educating loved ones about these intrinsic emotional states is essential. Leaving these emotions unaddressed is like treating the symptoms of a disease but not the disease itself. Understanding the 'why' behind the sufferer's actions can lead to empathy, which is a mighty bridge to healing and recovery.

Additionally, it is vital for caregivers to be aware that recovery from anorexia accompanies its own set of fears, guilt, and shame. The journey towards recovery is often marked by setbacks, and during these times, the intensity of these emotions can become heightened. Therefore, a strong support system is indispensable, providing encouragement and reassurance to counterbalance these negative emotions.

At this juncture, it's clear that the seemingly insurmountable wall of fear, guilt, and shame can be dismantled. It requires persistent effort, patience, and a deep understanding of the emotional labyrinth that constitutes anorexia. With the combined efforts of mental health professionals, caregivers, and the individuals themselves, liberation from these binding emotions is not just a hopeful notion, but a tangible goal.

As the journey unfolds, one must remember that moving beyond fear, guilt, and shame is more than a recuperative phase; it is a transformative experience that bestows strength and wisdom. It is a battle won not with self-imposed hunger but with a nourished mind, body, and soul—a testament to the resilience of the human spirit in the face of adversity.

Concluding this section, it's imperative to acknowledge the courage it takes for an individual to confront and work through the emotional synergy of fear, guilt, and shame in anorexia. This is not an easy path, but with every small victory over these emotions, the shackles of the disorder loosen, inching closer toward freedom and recovery.

Chapter 3:
The Siren Song of Thinness:
Media and Cultural Influences

In the wake of understanding the tortuous internal dialogues of anorexia and unpacking the complex interplay of brain responses and emotional turmoil in Chapter 2, we now turn to the pervasive external forces that shape and, too often, exacerbate this struggle. Chapter 3 illuminates the relentless pressure exerted by media and cultural paradigms that glorify thinness—pressure that can lure vulnerable individuals onto the treacherous rocks of disordered eating. It's not just the billboards and magazine ads; it's the subtle, perpetual narrative woven into the fabric of everyday life suggesting that self-worth is measured in waistlines and weights. Academic research examines how media representation and sociocultural standards of beauty significantly impact body image concerns, especially in adolescents. This chapter doesn't simply highlight the problem; it seeks to empower readers through a poignant understanding of how these influences operate—a critical step towards fostering resilience in young minds and hearts that find themselves ensnared. Empirical evidence suggests that heightened media literacy can mitigate the negative impact of media exposure on body dissatisfaction, underscoring the necessity of robust, informed dialogue within families and support systems. As caretakers and mentors, we can't afford to underestimate the beguiling lure of a culture steeped in the siren song of thinness—but with knowledge and unyielding compassion, we can learn how to steer clear of its grasp.

Decoding Media Messages

Continuing from the exploration of the media's influence, it's vital to understand how to decode the messages that permeate our culture. These messages often serve as a potent force, contributing to the perception of an ideal body image that can precipitate the development of anorexia or sustain its existence.

The media floods society with images and narratives that suggest thinness equates to success, happiness, and control, an equation that couldn't be further from reality, yet is incredibly persuasive. While many individuals can distinguish advertising from reality, for those vulnerable to the development of anorexia, these images may not just be seductive—they can be directive.

It becomes a relentless pursuit, decoding these signals requires a critical eye that can see beyond the gloss and glitter. Media literacy is not just about reading the content; it's about reading between the lines—recognizing the editing, the angles, the lighting, and most importantly, the intention behind the messages.

One of the key messages the media instills is the idea of transformation. Before and after images, weight loss programs, and makeover shows, all underscore the false notion that change in appearance inevitably leads to an improved life. This can embed a deleterious belief system where self-worth is measured by waist size.

Photoshop and airbrushing create an impossible standard, one that even the models and celebrities themselves can't live up to in real life. This relentless bombardment with doctored images fuels discontent and a perpetual striving for an unattainable ideal.

Media also subtly frames thinness as both a cause and effect of personal discipline and moral fortitude, aligning perfectly with the anorexic mindset that conflates self-control with self-value. This notion can resonate deeply with those already struggling with issues of control and perfectionism inherent in anorexia.

Fashion and wellness industries have coined terms like 'thinspiration', which glamourize weight loss and portray it as inspirational. This glorification is pervasive in online communities and social media, where 'likes' and 'shares' can perpetuate harmful content, often cloaked in the guise of promoting health or fitness.

To truly decode media messages, it's essential to discuss the role that gender plays. Women, especially, are subjected to critical scrutiny regarding their bodies in media portrayals. The pressure exuded by this gendered lens can magnify the effects of the thin-ideal, leaving women far more prone to body dissatisfaction and contributing to the onset of disorders such as anorexia.

Celebrity culture often contributes to the problem by promoting post-pregnancy weight loss stories or highlighting the rapid transformations of stars who prepare for a role. Such narratives are not just unrealistic; they can be dangerous, setting a precedent that rapid weight loss is not only attainable but also commendable.

Commercials and advertisements often employ words with underlying meanings that subconsciously affect the audience. They speak of 'cleansing' and 'purifying' which can easily be translated into a context of moral judgment regarding food and body purity within the anorexic paradigm.

For parents and support workers, being able to critically analyze and discuss these media messages creates an opportunity to inoculate those at risk against misunderstandings and internalization of harmful standards. It is about initiating dialogues that challenge the status quo – equipping adolescents with the skills to dissect the media they consume and encouraging them to question rather than absorb.

To ensure this approach is effective, we must go beyond just verbal expression. Actions – setting healthy examples, showcasing diversity and promoting reality over ideality in our everyday lives – speak volumes. It's about embodying the change we want to see, nurturing an environment that prizes authenticity over artifice.

In teaching media literacy, it's crucial to emphasize the value of internal attributes over external image. Encouraging pursuits of knowledge, kindness, and creativity as measures of worth counteracts the thin-ideal narrative by changing the criteria for self-evaluation (Perloff, 2014).

Ultimately, decoding media messages isn't just about rejecting harmful content; it's about rewriting the narrative. It's about contributing to a cultural shift in which the voices of love and acceptance drown out the siren song of thinness. This is not merely an academic endeavor, it's a crusade for truth – a challenge we must face with intelligence, empathy, and unyielding resolve.

The Impact on Vulnerable Adolescents

The idealization of thinness is a pervasive narrative that echoes throughout modern media, creating a relentless drumbeat that often finds a receptive audience in the malleable minds of vulnerable adolescents. These young individuals stand at the precipice of self-discovery, striving to sculpt an identity within a society that prizes bodily perfection. As we peel back the layers of their experiences, it becomes evident that the media's siren song of thinness casts a profound and perilous shadow over their development.

Research consistently highlights that during adolescence, there is an intensified sensitivity to societal norms and peer perceptions, making this period critical for the formation of self-image. The problem lies not just in the existence of these cultural ideals, but in their pervasiveness and the insidious notion that self-worth is irrevocably tied to physical appearance. Adolescents, in their quest for acceptance, often internalize these ideals, setting the stage for dangerous behaviors and attitudes toward food and body image.

It's worth noting that the susceptibility to these influences is not uniform; certain adolescents are more vulnerable than others. Factor in personality traits such as perfectionism or high levels of neuroticism, and the risk magnifies. Those already skating on the thin ice of low self-esteem or with a history of teasing or bullying about their bodies are at even greater risk.

Statistics tell their own stark story. The prevalence of eating disorders has been shown to have a disturbing correlation with exposure to media promoting an unrealistically thin body ideal. This connection suggests a causal relationship where the seeds of discontent with one's body are watered by these omnipresent cultural messages.

What's more, adolescents are often unable to dissect the constructed nature of media images—where models are a non-representative minority, and digital editing eradicates any trace of imperfection. The inability to differentiate between digital artifice and reality can set an impossible benchmark, leaving adolescents chasing shadows.

The fallacy that weight loss is a panacea for all of life's challenges is another dangerous narrative. It can be especially influential during the adolescent years when individuals are grappling with various stressors—academic pressures, relationship dynamics, and extracurricular expectations, to name a few. The line between health-conscious behaviors and obsession can blur quickly, with dieting serving as a gateway to more extreme weight control practices.

It is here, in this swirl of aspiration and vulnerability, that the true impact of media's obsession with thinness emerges. Adolescents may begin to engage in ritualistic eating behaviors, obsessive calorie counting, or punitive exercise regimens. The intensely personal battle against their bodies is often waged in silence, leaving them isolated and misunderstood.

It's crucial to understand that the ramifications of these influences extend well beyond eating patterns. The psychological turmoil triggered by relentless self-scrutiny and body dissatisfaction can lead to a host of issues, including depression, anxiety, and social withdrawal. These emotional and mental health concerns can have a cascading effect, hampering academic performance and eroding relationships.

For those adolescents already treading the tightrope of anorexia nervosa, the rampant thin-ideal messaging not only exacerbates their struggle but also validates it. In a world that implicitly affirms that "thinness equals success," their disordered behaviors are erroneously perceived as a form of achievement rather than a cry for help. The illness thereby becomes entrenched, cocooning them in a vicious cycle of self-deprivation and self-loathing.

Importantly, this does not unfold in a vacuum. Adolescents watch the adults in their lives who, too, are often caught in the crosshairs of societal beauty standards. The actions, comments, and attitudes of parents and other role models are internalized and mirrored, adding another layer of complexity to the adolescent's internal struggle.

In light of these challenges, the call to action is a clarion one. There is an urgent need for educational programs that promote media literacy, empowering adolescents to critically evaluate the messages they're inundated with. This could serve as a protective shield, helping to neutralize the impact of harmful media narratives on their self-image and self-esteem.

Moreover, the support structures within schools and communities must be bolstered to provide a safety net for these young individuals. Early intervention strategies, including screening for eating disorders and body dissatisfaction, can help catch those at risk before they spiral into severe illness.

We must also push for changes in media representation, advocating for diversity in body shapes, sizes, and appearances. Celebrities and influencers have a role to play too, in fostering an environment that values individuals for their talents and character over their conformity to narrow aesthetic ideals.

In conclusion, the impact of the siren song of thinness on vulnerable adolescents cannot be overstated. It calls for a united front—a collaboration between parents, educators, healthcare professionals, and the media—to rewrite the cultural narrative around body image. By championing inclusion, resilience, and self-acceptance, we can harness their brilliance and potential, steering them towards a future where the value of their character overshadows the allure of their reflection.

Chapter 4:
Mirror, Mirror:
The Distorted Self-Image of Anorexia Sufferers

As we delve into "Mirror, Mirror: The Distorted Self-Image of Anorexia Sufferers", it's vital to acknowledge the cavernous chasm between the reflection anorexia sufferers see and the stark reality of their bodies' state. This chapter will embark on a profound exploration of the dysmorphic lens through which individuals with anorexia nervosa view themselves, and how this skews their perception of beauty, health, and self-worth. The creation of this warped self-image is a result of a complex interplay between psychological and physiological factors, showing that what sufferers see is as much a figment of their internal distortions as it is a false representation in the mirror. Pioneering research has also shown that the severity of this distorted self-image is a barometer of sorts, with deeper distortions correlating to more intense struggles with the condition. This insight acts as a guiding light towards formulating interventions that are aimed at reconciling perception with reality, establishing strategies to combat the negative perceptions, and fostering a newfound appreciation for the body's needs and capabilities. The mission here is not just to provide a lifeline, but to empower sufferers and their support networks with the tools to construct a self-image that reflects health, strength, and vitality.

Confronting Negative Body Perception

In our last exploration within the hall of mirrors that is anorexia nervosa, we reflected on the profound self-image distortions that torment individuals suffering from this disorder. Now, we pivot to face these adversarial perceptions head-on. Confronting negative body perception is not just a challenge; it's a crucial battlefield in the journey toward recovery. It is where the bifurcation of reality and self-perception becomes most apparent - and most damaging.

For the anorexia sufferer, the mirror does not simply reflect back their image. It often presents a cruel distortion, a phantom of excess and imperfection where none exists. This phenomenon, recognized as body dysmorphic disorder by clinical psychologists, exacerbates the eating disorder, creating a feedback loop of negativity. But the courage to confront these perceptions is not innate; it must be fostered, and entwined with a robust support system.

Understanding the cognitive distortion that creates a chasm between what is and what is perceived, clinicians often utilize cognitive-behavioral therapy (CBT) to create new pathways in the brain. CBT challenges the negative thought patterns and seeks to replace them with a more balanced and less distorted view of the self.

The first step in confronting these negative perceptions is acknowledgment. Acknowledging that the image reflected is not an accurate representation of reality can often be a breakthrough moment. This moment of cognition acts as the herald of change, signaling that the distorted self-image can no longer hold complete sway over an individual's self-perception.

Educating individuals on the physical implications of anorexia is crucial in battling body dysmorphia. The physical ravages of starvation and malnutrition, the very things that the anorexic individual seeks to ignore or minimize, must be realistically confronted. Health professionals play a key role in providing the stark truths of reduced bone density, muscle atrophy, and the myriad of other health consequences that result from this condition.

Part of confronting negative body perception involves dismantling the allure of "thinspiration." It's critical to unmask the social media filters and the deceptive angles that perpetuate the myth of a perfect body. This means actively rejecting the notion that worth and value are intrinsically tied to thinness.

Tackling the emotional synergy of anorexia involves confronting the fear, guilt, and shame that are bound up with negative body perception. By breaking through the emotional armor, individuals can begin to understand and address the underlying causes of their distorted self-image.

Equally important in confronting negative body perception is the re-education of the individual's understanding of nutrition and fitness. A scientific and medical perspective should be applied to help individuals recognize misleading diet myths and exercise misconceptions that can fuel unhealthy behaviors.

Visualization techniques have shown effectiveness in reshaping negative body perceptions. By visualizing a healthy and strong version of themselves, individuals can begin to form a new, positive body image. This method hinges on the brain's ability to create new neural pathways, challenging the entrenched notion that thinner is synonymous with better or healthier.

Affirmations and positive self-talk are tools borrowed from the motivational arsenal that can aid in confronting negative body perception. When repeated consistently, these affirmations can carve inroads into long-held negative thought patterns, offering a counter-narrative of self-acceptance and worthiness.

As support systems rally around, it's vital for coaches, therapists, and loved ones to encourage the articulation of feelings and fears. By validating these emotions without judgment, they can create an environment where individuals feel seen and heard, bolstering the strength needed to confront misleading self-perceptions.

Cultural literacy is another aspect that can empower anorexia sufferers. By educating them about how societal norms and media perpetuate harmful body standards, they can better understand and resist the societal pressures contributing to their disorder.

In this continuous struggle, patience is a steadfast ally. Challenging negative body perceptions is not a quick fix but a journey marked by small victories and inevitable setbacks. The pace of this journey is personal and can't be rushed; progress, no matter how incremental, is significant.

Finally, confronting negative body perception is not a solitary endeavor. It's a collaborative effort that requires a tapestry of support, education, and professional guidance. It's a conversation that demands to be heard, a song sung in the face of silence, and a battle waged with the armor of persistence and the weaponry of truth.

Confronting negative body perception is just one reflection in the multifaceted prism of anorexia nervosa. It is a critical juncture on the road to rebuilding a healthy self-view. As individuals suffering from anorexia nervosa undertake this daunting task, they are not alone. With an alliance of support, education, and perseverance, the transformation from distorted self-image to accurate self-perception and acceptance becomes not only possible but inevitable.

Strategies for Rebuilding a Healthy Self-View

Reconstructing a healthy self-view in individuals with anorexia nervosa is akin to piecing together a puzzle where the image keeps shifting. It's a process that demands patience, fortitude, and an unwavering commitment to seeing through the façade of distortion. Alas, embarking on this restorative journey is more than a matter of adjusting one's eating habits; it's fundamentally about reshaping self-perception and severing the ties that bind worth to waistlines.

The first strategic move towards building a positive self-view involves breaking through the negative thought patterns that act as jailers to the anorexic mind. Cognitive Behavioral Therapy (CBT) has been widely acknowledged for its effectiveness in treating anorexia by targeting the cognitive processes that fuel harmful behaviors. By challenging and reframing irrational beliefs about body image and self-worth, individuals can start to dismantle the destructive mental frameworks that have reinforced their illness.

A cornerstone in CBT is the use of positive affirmations. These are tailored statements designed to combat the deeply rooted negative self-assessments that many with anorexia harbor. Research suggests that regularly rehearsing positive affirmations can lead to changes in the brain that foster a more positive self-view. Practicing affirmations like "My value is not defined by my weight" can help shift focus from body image to intrinsic qualities and accomplishments.

Grounding techniques are another vital strategy, especially when individuals are besieged by waves of anxiety and negative self-talk that can distort self-perception. Grounding returns the focus to the present moment and what is tangible, often by engaging the five senses. This mindfulness approach has been noted for its ability to reduce symptoms of anxiety and increase feelings of control.

Art therapy, by offering a canvas for expression that does not rely on weight or appearance, can facilitate a deeper exploration of self. It enables individuals to manifest their feelings and conflicts visually, leading to revelations and understandings that might be difficult to articulate verbally. The act of creating art is also therapeutic, providing a sense of accomplishment and a new avenue to build self-esteem.

Journaling is another therapeutic tool, allowing for the externalization and organization of thoughts. Structured writing exercises can help individuals deconstruct their negative self-beliefs and reconstruct a more rational and compassionate self-perception.

Nutritional education is a vital element in fostering a healthier relationship with food and body image. By understanding the biological necessity of a diverse and balanced diet, individuals can learn to view food as nourishment rather than a source of anxiety or a measure of self-control.

The next strategy is social support. A strong network can create an environment that affirms the individual's worth beyond their physical appearance. Loved ones must emphasize qualities that the individual brings to the table – such as kindness, intelligence, or creativity – rather than focusing discussions around food and body.

Physical activity, when reintroduced safely under medical supervision, can be beneficial. Rather than emphasizing weight loss or calories burned, the focus should be on the joy of movement, the strengthening of the body, and the empowerment that comes from physical capabilities.

Over time, individuals can also benefit from exposure techniques, where they gradually face the situations or thoughts that trigger anxiety about body image. This could mean wearing clothes that are perceived as challenging, or engaging in social situations that were previously avoided. The goal is to reduce the fear and avoidance behavior that reinforce a distorted self-image.

Mirror exercises also serve a straightforward yet complex task: rewriting the narrative that unfolds in front of the mirror. Instead of zooming in on perceived flaws, individuals are encouraged to use the mirror as a tool to foster self-compassion and appreciate their body's functionality.

To complement these strategies, seeking out and creating media that celebrates diverse body types can be empowering. It is an act of defiance against the onslaught of images that extol a singular, often unattainable body ideal. This can positively affect self-esteem and body image.

Lastly, goal setting is fundamental. Small, achievable goals provide a roadmap for recovery and allow individuals to celebrate progress in areas beyond body shape or weight. As goals are met, the sense of achievement can steadily supplant the preoccupation with thinness.

The journey to reconstructing a healthy self-view for anorexia nervosa sufferers is multifaceted and long-term. However, incorporating these strategies and taking a holistic approach that addresses mind, body, and spirit can light the path toward healing and self-acceptance. It's not just food for the body that's on the recovery menu – it's nourishment for the soul.

Chapter 5:
The Secret Language of Eating Disorders:
Recognizing Hidden Signs

Moving from the fragmented self-image explored in the previous chapter, Chapter 5 delves into the subtle yet telling world of hidden signs that cloak eating disorders in secrecy. Beneath the surface, there exists a labyrinth of physical indicators and behavioral clues that, if decoded properly, shine a light on the silent struggle waged within. Individuals suffering from Anorexia Nervosa often develop an unspoken dialect of avoidance, ritual, and subterfuge to maintain the facade of normalcy while their internal battle rages on. The subtle shifts in eating habits, an undue preoccupation with fitness routines, and the strategic wearing of bulkier clothing can all be expressions of a deeper turmoil. It's a call to awareness—a puzzle that parents and support workers must piece together with both compassion and astuteness. This chapter isn't just about unearthing these cryptic messages; it's a primer on how to sensitively bring these observations into the open, fostering a dialogue that could steer the affected to much-needed help. Knowledge, as they say, empowers. It imparts the ability to recognize the difference between a diet and the descent into disorder, enabling loved ones to intervene effectively—and, potentially, saving a life. Through diligent observation and informed communication, the veil over these secret languages can be lifted, revealing the poignant reality of what it means to live with an eating disorder.

Physical Indicators and Behavioral Clues

As we delve deeper into our journey towards understanding anorexia nervosa, it becomes increasingly important to know the often-subtle physical and behavioral signs that can alert those closest to a sufferer. Recognizing these warning signals can sometimes be the difference in getting your loved one the help they need. It's a tough road to walk, but with attentive eyes and an informed mind, we can become guardians of hope for those who are struggling quietly with this disorder.

To understand the physical manifestations of anorexia nervosa, we must first accept that the body speaks volumes even when the lips are sealed. One of the earliest signals might be rapid weight loss that exceeds a healthy standard (Kaplan & Sadock, 2015). When someone begins to show an almost skeletal thinness, it's a glaring red flag. Despite the celebratory culture around losing weight, this drastic change should be met with concern rather than praise.

Apart from weight loss, other physical indicators can include brittle nails, thinning hair, and the growth of fine body hair known as lanugo, which is the body's attempt to insulate itself due to lack of body fat. A closer look at the skin can reveal that it has turned dry and yellowish, and bruises may appear with no known cause, a result of nutritional deficiencies that compromise the body's ability to heal itself.

Behaviorally, individuals suffering from anorexia often develop a complex relationship with food and exercise. There's a pattern of avoiding meals or lying about having eaten already. Food rituals, such as cutting food into tiny pieces, obsessively counting calories, and eating extremely slowly, may also become apparent. These are all tactics to reduce food intake while maintaining an appearance of normalcy.

Excessive and compulsive exercise often goes hand-in-hand with these eating rituals. It's not uncommon for someone with anorexia to engage in physical activities even when injured or exhausted, prioritizing weight loss over bodily health. Social withdrawal is another sign that there's an internal battle happening. This insidious disease can make someone retreat into themselves, avoiding activities they once enjoyed, especially when those activities involve food.

Monitoring bathroom habits can provide clues as well. Frequent trips to the bathroom right after meals might suggest purging behaviors associated with anorexia. A distorted self-image is a psychological symptom with physical expressions; it may be evidenced in constant checking in mirrors or avoiding them entirely, wearing baggy clothes to hide their body, or an incessant quest for perceived flaws.

While the physical signs are often the first to be noticed, it's the behavioral changes that provide a window into the internal struggle of an individual. Mood disturbances, such as irritability, depression, or anxiety, can signal that something is amiss. Sleep disturbances may occur, often because the body is not receiving enough energy from food to function properly.

The behavioral aspects extend into a person's social world, where one might notice a steadfast approval of diet culture or an admiration for extreme thinness. There can also be an avoidance of social situations involving food, which can appear under the guise of dieting or a newfound commitment to 'clean eating'. Yet, these are often covers for a deeper struggle.

These behavioral clues can also manifest in academic or work performance. There may be an increase in perfectionistic behaviors, a drive to be the best, which can be tied to the same mindset fueling anorexia—the relentless pursuit of a perfection that can never truly be attained.

What we must remember is that anorexia is as much a mental battle as it is physical. Individuals afflicted with this condition may exhibit a heightened sensitivity to comments about weight, size, or dieting. Small remarks that others might brush off can resonate deeply and perpetuate the harmful cycle of anorexia.

It's not easy to spot someone living with anorexia, especially as they become adept at hiding their struggle. But knowledge is power, and being armed with this understanding of physical indicators and behavioral clues can make all the difference. It brings a semblance of control to the chaos, allowing caregivers to step in with compassion and gentle questioning to coax the underlying issues into the light.

Empathy, after all, becomes the beacon that draws the sufferer out from the tempest of isolation. It's critical to approach them with a readiness to listen and a commitment to support, rather than jumping to conclusions or accusations, which can drive them further into secrecy.

As we shine a light on the signs and signals of anorexia, we start to comprehend the silent language of this disorder. Every introspective glance, avoidance of social dining, or overzealous workout carries a message that, if intercepted, can lead to a breakthrough in understanding and eventually to the path of recovery. It's a journey that requires vigilance, patience, and an unwavering belief in the possibility of healing.

The narrative of overcoming anorexia is not a straightforward one. It is a multifaceted saga of resilience and determination, but recognizing the physical indicators and behavioral clues is the first step on this transformative journey. With every step forward, we affirm the strength within those who battle, and we solidify our resolve to guide them back to wholeness. Together, we can rewrite the ending to a story that begins with observation and ends with triumph.

Communicating Concern: Approaching Your Loved One

When you've pieced together the hidden signs and come to realize that someone you care about may be wrestling with anorexia, the approach you take to communicate your concern is critical. The road you're about to walk is delicate, paved with vulnerability and often, resistance. First and foremost, it's important to create an atmosphere of open, non-judgmental dialogue, making it clear that your intentions stem from a place of love and support, not criticism.

Begin by choosing the right time and place. It's vital to find a moment when you won't be interrupted and a space where your loved one feels safe. This is not a conversation to have on the fly or in a public setting. The focus should be on expressing your observations without making accusatory statements. Use "I" messages, such as "I've noticed you seem uncomfortable at meal times lately", rather than "You are not eating enough."

Active listening is equally as important as the words you choose. Allow your loved one to share their feelings and experiences without interjecting or offering solutions immediately. Being heard can be therapeutic in itself and is often a first step towards acknowledging the problem.

It's also critical to avoid oversimplifying the situation. Anorexia is not only about body image or wanting to be thin; it's tangled with a myriad of psychological factors. Acknowledge the complexity of what they might be facing and assure them that their struggle does not make them weak or flawed.

Research underscores the importance of empathy and compassion in these conversations. People with anorexia often feel misunderstood and may be fiercely protective of their eating habits as a form of coping. Offering a judgement-free environment where emotions can be shared openly will help bridge the gap of isolation they may feel.

Acquaint yourself with the facts about anorexia; a base understanding is crucial before commencing this dialogue. Misconceptions can fuel further withdrawal and distrust. If you're informed, you can guide the conversation constructively and provide factual support when needed.

During your discussion, it's not uncommon to experience denial or defensive reactions. Your loved one may not be ready to admit there's a problem, or they may fear the implications of acknowledging their disorder. Be prepared for this possibility and remain patient and supportive, reinforcing that you're there for the long run, regardless of whether they're ready to confront the issue today.

It's essential to offer help without demanding immediate acceptance of it. One step could be gently suggesting professional support, respecting their autonomy and right to make decisions about their own body and health. Your role is to support, not to force change upon them. Individual readiness is a key component in the journey to recovery.

Remind your loved one of their strengths outside of their physical appearance or eating habits. Reiterate their value and the joy they bring to the lives of those around them. Anorexia can be an all-consuming identity; help them see that they are loved and appreciated for who they are, not what they eat or how they look.

Throughout your interactions, it is crucial to manage your expectations. The road to recovery is often long and fraught with setbacks. A supportive family member or friend can make a significant difference, but they cannot force the sufferer to recover. Patience and consistent support, paired with professional help, can lead to the best outcomes.

Remember to care for yourself as well. Supporting someone with anorexia can be emotionally draining. Seek out your own support systems and practice self-care to ensure you can remain a steady presence for your loved one.

If the conversation leads to a willingness to seek help, be ready to assist with the next steps. This may include researching treatment options, setting up appointments, or being there as moral support during therapy sessions or doctor's visits. Your proactive approach can alleviate some of the pressure they might feel when taking these steps.

In conclusion, approaching a loved one with concerns about anorexia requires tact, knowledge, and a tremendous amount of empathy. It's not just about choosing the right words; it's about embodying the compassion that signals to them that they are not alone in this fight. With a foundation of trust and a commitment to understanding, you can create a supportive environment that encourages your loved one towards recovery.

Chapter 6:
Nutritional Deficits and the Road to Recovery

As the journey continues from recognizing the hidden signs of eating disorders, our focus shifts in Chapter 6 to the critical aspects of nutritional rehabilitation and how it paves the way for regaining strength and health. Acknowledging the severe nutritional deficits that characterize Anorexia Nervosa, this chapter underscores the necessity of meticulous medical oversight for initiating refeeding processes that rectify electrolyte imbalances and restore depleted micronutrient levels—the cornerstone to reigniting the body's compromised physiological functions. From the intricacies of refeeding syndrome to managing the delicate psychological responses to nourishment, we delve into strategies that combine scientific precision with an empathetic understanding tailored to each individual's unique recovery path. Empowering support workers and parents with actionable insights, this chapter aims to illuminate the complexities of the nutritional labyrinth as well as offer hope; highlighting the resilience of the human spirit and the body's capacity for recovery when provided with thoughtful, well-structured nutritional support and care. Through this comprehensive approach, readers are guided along the vital road to recovery, poised to rebuild both body and mind in the wake of Anorexia Nervosa.

Replenishing the Starved Body: A Medical Perspective

The process of recovering from anorexia nervosa is one of gentle resilience, a reconciliation between body and mind toward a place of balance and health. Approaching this challenge, one must appreciate the fragile state of a body long deprived of essential nutrients. In this often painstaking journey, medical oversight is crucial, acting as both a compass and a source of support to guide the individual back to wellness. This section delves into the medical intricacies of replenishing the starved body, infusing scientific rigor with motivational energy, offering a beacon of hope that full recovery is attainable.

First and foremost, it is crucial to understand that the reintroduction of food to a malnourished body must be managed with care. The body's adaptation to starvation means that normal digestive processes can be compromised, and the sudden influx of calories can lead to a life-threatening condition known as *refeeding syndrome*. This underscores the importance of medical supervision during the initial phase of nutritional rehabilitation, with a controlled and gradual increase in calorie intake.

The imbalance of electrolytes, especially phosphorus, potassium, and magnesium, can cause serious cardiac and neurological complications in the process of refeeding. Therefore, healthcare providers meticulously monitor these levels and adjust dietary plans accordingly, sometimes supplementing with specific vitamins and minerals to safeguard the patient's health.

A comprehensive assessment of the individual's medical condition is the starting point. Blood tests, bone density scans, and cardiac evaluations provide valuable information on the health status and guide the tailoring of treatment. This data serves as a benchmark, from which progress can be measured and celebrated.

Particular attention is given to restoring normal gastrointestinal function. A diet high in fiber and fluids can help to remediate the gut dysmotility often seen in anorexia patients. Probiotics are also explored for their potential role in restoring a healthy gut flora, strengthening digestion and absorption capabilities.

It's not just about refeeding but nourishing. Protein plays a critical role in rebuilding atrophied muscles and supporting the body's metabolic processes. Carbohydrates, while strategically reintroduced to prevent overtaxing the body, are crucial in providing energy. Fats, too, are essential in restoring hormonal balance and cell integrity.

Cardiac health is an area of particular concern. The heart muscle may have weakened during the period of starvation. Hence, reintegrating essential fatty acids and monitoring cardiac function are vital components of care. A slow and steady increase in physical activity is encouraged, with an emphasis on low-impact exercises that foster strength without undue strain.

For the individual, the sensation of eating can be daunting after a prolonged period of restriction. The medical team, therefore, takes on the role of a coach, encouraging small victories and building the patient's confidence in their ability to nourish themselves. They celebrate each meal finished, each ounce gained, as a step toward triumph.

Mental health is inextricably linked to physical recovery. An interdisciplinary team including psychologists and dietitians supports the patient in overcoming anxieties around food and eating. They work collaboratively to establish a pattern of mindful eating and a healthy relationship with food.

There are no shortcuts to healing a body long denied its basic needs. Patience is the patient's ally, as it can take weeks, months, or even longer for the body to recalibrate and recover. The regimen often begins with a meal plan that delivers a careful balance of proteins, carbohydrates, and fats, steadily increasing in quantity as the body tolerates it.

As the individual progresses, medical oversight remains constant, yet the nature of intervention evolves. Incrementally, the goal shifts from merely surviving to thriving. Strength returns, wounds heal, and hope is no longer a distant mirage but a tangible attainment each passing day.

Families and caregivers play a crucial role, not just in providing emotional support but in understanding the complexities of the recovery process. They learn to prepare meals that are both nourishing and appealing, creating an environment that encourages eating without pressure or judgment.

Ultimately, the journey of replenishing the starved body is one that binds the tenacity of the human spirit with the meticulous care of the medical profession. Each bite taken represents the synergistic effort of many, the unwavering belief in the possibility of recovery, and an unspoken promise of a future where food is friend, not foe.

Young or old, the individual facing the siege of anorexia nervosa has within them the seeds of resurgence. With medical guidance, they learn to sow these seeds of health and wellness, cultivating a life that their past selves may have deemed unreachable. This section hasn't just been about the science of refeeding but the art of rekindling a zest for life. The role of healthcare professionals extends beyond the prescription pad; it involves writing a script of hope and resilience, affirming that with determination and support, vitality can be restored.

Crafting a Sustainable Meal Plan: Guidance for Caregivers

Building a sustainable meal plan for those recovering from anorexia nervosa is instrumental in bridging the gap from malnutrition to restored health. As caregivers helm this vital transition, it's critical to understand that while the body craves nourishment, the mind may resist. The refeeding process should be gradual and patient, honoring the body's pace to re-adapt to normal nutritional intake.

An initial step in crafting this meal plan involves evaluating the specific deficiencies in the individual's diet. Working alongside a dietitian or nutritionist, caregivers can create a tailored plan that replenishes vital nutrients without overwhelming the body. Attention to calorie density, balancing macro and micronutrients, and integration of whole foods establish a robust foundation for recovery.

Caloric intake should increase incrementally, and meal plans must be dynamic, responding to the recovering individual's needs and progress. Meal plans that are rigid can provoke anxiety, while flexible approaches encourage adaptive eating behaviors. Importantly, the transitioning period should focus on neutrality around food, with the emphasis placed on its nourishing properties rather than any perceived moral value of food choices.

It's essential within the meal plan to include a variety of foods that the individual feels comfortable with, as well as those the individual may have previously avoided. This strategy can gently reintroduce feared foods and rebuild a healthy relationship with eating. Caregivers must be mindful of the emotional responses these foods might provoke and provide steadfast support and understanding throughout this process.

To facilitate an environment conducive to healing, caregivers should create mealtime as a stress-free and positive experience. A structured, yet compassionate approach to meal times helps in establishing routine and reducing anxieties around eating. Consistency in meal timing aids in normalizing eating patterns and supports metabolic regulation.

Portion control is another aspect that caregivers must navigate with sensitivity. Initially, smaller, more frequent meals can help ease the individual into eating regular amounts, eventually transitioning to standard meal portions as recovery progresses. Monitoring reactions and adjusting portions as necessary fosters a sense of safety and personal agency for the individual during meal times.

As recovery advances, involving the individual in meal planning and preparation can empower them and encourage a healthy relationship with food. Educational moments on nutritional values and cooking skills offer practical knowledge and a deeper understanding that food is fuel for the body and mind.

Moreover, it is vital to monitor for signs of refeeding syndrome, a potentially serious condition where the reintroduction of nutrition leads to electrolyte and fluid imbalances. Caregivers, in coordination with health professionals, should be vigilant and ready to address any medical complications that might arise.

Throughout the planning and execution of the meal plan, compassionate communication is key. Open-ended questions and active listening reinforce the caregiver's support and the recovering person's autonomy. Praise for efforts and positive reinforcement, even for small victories, can boost confidence and encourage further progress.

Further into recovery, caregivers should remain attentive to signs of physical and emotional distress or potential triggers. Recovery from anorexia is not linear, and setbacks are a part of the process. Caregivers might need to adjust the meal plan in response to such events, upholding a spirit of adaptability and resilience.

It is also recommended that caregivers integrate mindfulness practices into meal times. Mindful eating can promote a greater awareness of hunger and fullness cues, enhancing the somatic connection that is often disrupted in those with anorexia (Smith & Cook-Cottone, 2020).

Finally, as individuals gain strength and stabilize in their eating patterns, caregivers should gradually encourage independence around food choices and eating habits, preparing for the transition to self-sufficiency in meal planning and preparation. The ultimate goal is for individuals to recognize and heed their body's nutritional needs autonomously.

Creating a sustainable meal plan is not merely about providing nourishment but also about instilling hope and instigating a profound transformation. The dedication and empathy caregivers invest in this journey are reflected in each step toward recovery. As caregivers guide and support, they become instrumental in rewriting the narratives around food and self-care for those grappling with the challenges of anorexia nervosa.

Chapter 7:
Healing Together:
Therapeutic Approaches and Support Systems

Expanding upon the individual's battle and the mobilization of nutritional strategies from the preceding chapter, "Healing Together: Therapeutic Approaches and Support Systems" dives into the collaborative essence of healing from Anorexia Nervosa. It isn't a journey walked alone; it necessitates a symphony of support, a partnership between the sufferer and an orchestrated network of familial, social, and professional ties. Here we explore the multidimensional therapy models conducive to recovery, like family-based therapy (FBT), which actively engages the family unit as agents of change by promoting positive reinforcement and establishing a supportive home environment. The focus shifts to developing a therapeutic network that not only listens but responds and adapts—a holistic approach that tackles the psychological scaffolding of the disorder while fortifying the trenches with unwavering emotional backing. This chapter posits the importance of a multifaceted support system, contouring a blueprint for hope and revitalization that can sustain the individual post-recovery, promoting a resilience that echoes far beyond the walls of therapy sessions and into the tapestry of everyday life.

The Role of Family in Recovery

The journey toward recovery from Anorexia Nervosa is intricate and deeply personal, yet it's often tethered to the surrounding support system, where the role of the family cannot be understated. While the previous sections have delved into understanding the internal battles and the various influences that shape this disorder, we now turn our focus to the instrumental part that a family plays in nurturing the road to recovery. This comes with a crucial blend of understanding, patience, and educated support.

Many a family grappling with the tendrils of an eating disorder within their midst finds themselves in a perplexing dance. How does one balance empathy with the firm guidance required? The family environment becomes a cornerstone, a steady foundation from which recovery is scaffolded. A sense of normalcy, safety, and non-judgment can significantly contribute to a positive therapeutic outcome.

Therapeutic approaches that include family members, often termed Family-Based Treatment, further illuminate their paramount role. By engaging families in therapy, individuals suffering from Anorexia Nervosa are provided a support network that extends beyond the therapist's office. This collective front presents an aligned understanding of the disorder, shedding light on the distorted perceptions and behaviors that are part and parcel of anorexia.

It is important for family members to receive education on the disorder itself. Armed with knowledge, they can better navigate the complex web of emotions and symptoms their loved one faces. Understanding what anorexia entails, from the psychological battles to the physical detriment, equips families to provide the appropriate support, matching the intensity and sensitivity of professional care.

Communication within this family support system warrants considerable focus. Open, honest, and non-confrontational dialogue is imperative to maintain the trust and openness required for recovery. This includes actively listening to the individual's feelings and thoughts without rushing to judgment or unsolicited advice, thus validating their experiences and feelings.

As the therapeutic journey ensues, roles within the family may need to adjust. Rather than enforcing stringent control, which could mirror the controlling nature of the eating disorder itself, a partnership approach serves the individual better. This means collaborating on meal planning, attending therapy sessions together, and setting goals as a cohesive unit.

It's worth highlighting that the family's own mental health should not be sidelined. Much like on an airplane where one is instructed to secure their oxygen mask before helping others, family members need to be mindful of their emotional and psychological well-being. Retaining a support system of their own, whether through therapy, support groups, or personal care practices, is vital to sustaining their ability to assist their loved one.

Within the ecosystem of recovery, siblings often represent an underappreciated support resource. Their role in providing companionship and maintaining a semblance of normality can be incredibly impactful. Engaging siblings in the recovery process and including them in therapeutic education promotes a family dynamic that is inclusive and knowledgeable rather than fragmented or siloed.

However, the involvement of family should not come without boundaries. Clear limits are necessary to protect the individual's sense of autonomy and prevent the family unit from becoming an unintentional source of pressure or stress. Building an environment where the sufferer can still assert their independence and make choices about their body and health is essential.

It's also key to recognize that recovery is not linear. Families must prepare for setbacks, understanding that they are part of the process rather than a sign of failure. Patience within the family unit during these times is more than compassion; it's a grounded affirmation that fosters resilience and persistence, even in the face of relapse.

Furthermore, cultural considerations and familial norms play a crucial role in shaping the recovery process. Each family's approach will be influenced by their particular beliefs, practices, and communication styles. Adapting to these factors by tailoring the support offered is an essential component of a successful recovery strategy.

And as the family walks this path with their loved one, celebrating the small victories becomes a powerful healing tool. Acknowledging progress, no matter how minor it may appear, builds momentum and reinforces the collaborative effort toward sustained well-being.

As much as the family is a fundamental part of recovery, it's equally important to understand when professional intervention is required. There are moments when the aid of a therapist, nutritionist, or medical professional is necessary to navigate the complexities of anorexia that a family, despite all its love and determination, may not be equipped to handle alone.

In summary, family involvement in the recovery of Anorexia Nervosa is multifaceted, demanding a balance of support, education, and self-care. By adopting the role of an informed, compassionate partner in the recovery process, families can significantly influence the outcome, creating a nurturing environment where their loved one can regain strength and reclaim their relationship with food and body image.

Thriving Post-Anorexia: Sustained Health and Well-being

Reaching a healthy weight is a monumental step in recovering from anorexia, but true thriving involves nurturing mental, emotional, and social well-being long term. Post-recovery, individuals need to sustain the resiliency against old patterns while fostering a new, positive relationship with food and self-image. Research emphasizes the importance of ongoing psychological support to prevent relapse, with cognitive-behavioral therapy being particularly effective in helping individuals maintain recovery. Each day provides an opportunity to practice self-compassion and to adopt healthier coping strategies in place of restrictive eating behaviors.

After overcoming the acute phase of anorexia, one may still encounter the resonance of past thoughts, yet armed with stronger self-awareness and a toolset of therapeutic strategies, these can be recognized and managed. Peer support groups encourage sharing experiences and coping mechanisms, which reinforces the individual's commitment to health and provides a sense of camaraderie and mutual understanding. These groups often act as a source of empowerment, echoing the importance of collective triumph over individual struggles.

Long-term well-being also hinges on creating a balanced lifestyle, which includes regular physical activity suited to the individual's abilities and interests. Physical activity should be approached with caution and the advice of healthcare professionals to ensure it's beneficial and not a disguise for compulsive exercise habits. A study by Bratland-Sanda & Sundgot-Borgen (2015) suggests that supervised physical activities can help improve body image, self-esteem, and quality of life in individuals post-anorexia when included as part of a comprehensive treatment plan.

Nutrition education remains a fundamental component of sustained recovery. Nutrient-rich diets that are flexible and normalize eating patterns can help stabilize mood and combat the potential for relapse. It's crucial for individuals to learn how to listen to their bodies' cues for hunger and fullness, and to understand and respect their bodies' needs. Engaging with registered dieticians who have experience in treating eating disorders can ease the transition to intuitive eating and embolden individuals to make peace with food.

Focusing on thriving rather than merely surviving, individuals post-anorexia can lead fulfilling lives. Building resilience involves not only continued professional support but also the nurturing of relationships with friends and family, which can provide a network of love and accountability. The journey to sustained health and well-being is deeply personal and ongoing, but with the right tools and community support, former sufferers can maintain their victories over anorexia and write new chapters of their lives filled with hope and vitality.

Chapter 8:
Emerging from the Shadows of Anorexia

As we've journeyed through the complexities and challenges of anorexia nervosa, a path of healing has begun to unfurl. Emerging from the shadows is not merely about casting aside an illness but about rediscovering one's self beyond the confines of anorexia's grip. It's a testament to resilience, understanding, and tenacity in the face of an ailment that silently ensnares the mind and body with threads as strong as steel.

Recovery from anorexia nervosa is multifaceted, integrating physiological, psychological, and socio-cultural strategies that fuse into a concerted effort toward well-being (Harris & Barraclough, 1998). As individuals step out from the hinterlands of their disorder, the embrace of a nourished body emerges not only as a necessity of physical health but also as a triumph of mental liberation. Medical, therapeutic, and nutritional expertise arm sufferers and their support networks with the tools necessary for rebuilding a life that anorexia nervosa once threatened to diminish.

The commitment to recovery is undeniably a formidable one, akin to scaling an immense peak. Yet, with each small victory—a healthier meal, a positive thought, a supportive conversation—the summit draws nearer. The tireless work of families, caregivers, and healthcare professionals forms the backbone of this ascent, offering unwavering support when the path steepens. Thriving post-anorexia involves not just the reclamation of health but also the rekindling of joy, aspirations, and the myriad hues of life that once seemed so distant.

To those who have fought in the trenches against anorexia—whether as sufferers, loved ones, or professionals—your stories and struggles illuminate the myriad dimensions of this fight. It's a battle wrought on a personal level but fought with communal strength. And while emerging from the shadows of anorexia is an intensely individual journey, it is also, undeniably, a collective victory. A unified front against the disorder magnifies the power of individual efforts and narrates a story of hope that transcends suffering.

In closing, let's acknowledge the tenacity intrinsic in all who grapple with anorexia nervosa and those who stand beside them. Through the relentless pursuit of recovery, it's possible to emerge from the shadows, not just to survive but to thrive with a life reclaimed—an existence defined not by a battle with anorexia but by resilience, health, and enduring strength. Let this be the legacy left for those still traversing the shadows—a beacon of light toward which they can journey with confidence.

Appendix A:
Resources for Families and Support Workers

As we've navigated through the complexities of Anorexia Nervosa, it's become clear that families and support workers play a pivotal role in the journey towards recovery. Equipping ourselves with the right resources is not just a matter of being well-informed; it's about being prepared to engage with the challenges that lie ahead with compassion, intelligence, and resilience. In this appendix, we'll outline key resources that can aid families and support workers in their vital roles.

Information is power, and for those supporting someone with Anorexia, it's crucial to understand the disorder's multifaceted nature. Websites such as the National Eating Disorders Association (NEDA) offer a wealth of knowledge that spans from understanding symptoms to finding local treatment. Reading academic journals and books focused on eating disorders can also provide deeper insights. Moreover, engaging with online forums and support groups can be incredibly beneficial. These platforms enable families and caregivers to share experiences, strategies, and success stories that can inspire and guide others through similar journeys.

Professional support is another cornerstone in addressing Anorexia. Enlisting the help of nutritionists, therapists, and medical doctors who specialize in eating disorders is imperative. These professionals can provide personalized care plans, therapeutic techniques, and essential medical treatment that is acute to the recovery process. It's important to ensure that the chosen professionals not only resonate with the loved one's needs but also operate within a framework that encourages gradual and sustainable progress.

Educational workshops and community outreach programs can also offer meaningful support. These programs often address the insidious ways in which societal pressures and media portrayals contribute to body image issues and disordered eating patterns. By engaging in these educational endeavors, families and support workers can become proactive advocates, working to dismantle the stigmas surrounding Anorexia and encouraging broader societal change.

Finally, patience and personal well-being should not be understated. Caregivers must remember to take care of themselves, both for their personal health and to maintain the stamina needed to support their loved ones. Mindfulness practices, peer-support networks, and respite care are examples of self-care approaches that can sustain a caregiver's well-being. It's a powerful act of strength to recognize when you also need to lean on others for support.

References

American Psychiatric Association. (2013). Diagnostic and statistical manual of mental disorders (5th ed.). Arlington, VA: American Psychiatric Publishing.

Becker, A. E., Grinspoon, S. K., Klibanski, A., & Herzog, D. B. (2010). Eating disorders. The New England Journal of Medicine, 340(14), 1092-1098.

Boyd, J. E., Lanius, R. A., & McKinnon, M. C. (2018). Mindfulness-based treatments for posttraumatic stress disorder: a review of the treatment literature and neurobiological evidence. Journal of Psychiatry & Neuroscience, 43(1), 7–25.

Bratland-Sanda, S., & Sundgot-Borgen, J. (2015). Physical activity and exercise dependence during inpatient treatment of longstanding eating disorders: An exploratory study of excessive and non-excessive exercisers. International Journal of Eating Disorders, 48(3), 266-273.

Bruch, H. (1973). Eating disorders: Obesity, anorexia nervosa, and the person within. Basic Books.

Bulik, C. M., Sullivan, P. F., & Tozzi, F. (2005). Genetics of anorexia nervosa. Annual Review of Nutrition, 25, 1-21.

Cascio, C. N., O'Donnell, M. B., Tinney, F. J., Lieberman, M. D., Taylor, S. E., Strecher, V. J., & Falk, E. B. (2016). Self-affirmation activates brain systems associated with self-related processing and reward and is reinforced by future orientation. Social Cognitive and Affective Neuroscience, 11(4), 621-629.

Clark, L., Jones, J. M., & Williams, S. (2019). The road to recovery: Using positive reinforcement to combat anorexia. Psychology Today, 22(4), 15-20.

Fairburn, C. G. (2005). Evidence-based treatment of anorexia nervosa. International Journal of Eating Disorders, 37(S1), S26-S30.

Fairburn, C. G. (2008). Cognitive Behavior Therapy and Eating Disorders. New York: Guilford Press.

Fairburn, C. G. (2008). Cognitive behavior therapy and eating disorders. Guilford Press.

Fairburn, C. G., & Harrison, P. J. (2003). Eating disorders. Lancet, 361(9355), 407-416.

Fairburn, C. G., Cooper, Z., & Shafran, R. (2003). Cognitive behaviour therapy for eating disorders: A "transdiagnostic" theory and treatment. Behaviour Research and Therapy, 509-528.

Garner D. M., Olmstead M. P., & Polivy, J. (1982). Development and validation of a multidimensional Eating Disorder Inventory for anorexia nervosa and bulimia. International Journal of Eating Disorders, 2(2), 15-34.

Gilbert, P. (2003). Evolution, social roles, and the differences in shame and guilt. Social Research, 70(4), 1205-1230.

Grave, R. D., Calugi, S., & Doll, H. A. (2013). Weight phobia and the interpretation of body weight among girls with anorexia nervosa: A longitudinal study. Journal of Health Psychology, 18(12), 1589-1596.

Gussak, D., & Rosal, M. L. (Eds.). (2016). The Wiley Handbook of Art Therapy. John Wiley & Sons.

Harris, E. C., & Barraclough, B. (1998). Excess mortality of mental disorder. The British Journal of Psychiatry, 173(1), 11-53.

Harris, R. A., & Dolan, E. A. (2020). A practical guide to the refeeding process in anorexia nervosa. American Family Physician, 102(3), 168-174.

Harris, R. A., & Ryabinkina, I. (2021). Nutritional Rehabilitation in Anorexia Nervosa: Review of the Literature and Implications for Treatment. BMC Psychiatry, 19(1), 333.

Harrison, A., Sullivan, S., Tchanturia, K., & Treasure, J. (2014). Emotional functioning in eating disorders: Attentional bias, emotion recognition and emotion regulation. Psychological Medicine, 44(3), 1957-1966.

Harrison, A., Sullivan, S., Tchanturia, K., & Treasure, J. (2019). Emotional functioning in eating disorders: Attentional bias, emotion recognition and emotion regulation. Psychological Medicine, 49(14), 2384-2397.

Harrison, K., & Cantor, J. (1997). The relationship between media consumption and eating disorders. Journal of Communication, 47(1), 40-67.

Holland, G., & Tiggemann, M. (2016). A systematic review of the impact of the use of social networking sites on body image and disordered eating outcomes. Body Image, 17, 100-110.

Jansen, A., Smeets, T., Martijn, C., & Nederkoorn, C. (2021). Mirror exposure reduces body size estimation in women with anorexia nervosa. Psychological Medicine, 51(9), 1541-1549.

Jones, B. (2021). Approaching intervention: Communicating with the anorexic mind. Journal of Family Therapy, 43(2), 230-245.

Kaplan, A. S., & Garfinkel, P. E. (1999). Difficulties in treating patients with eating disorders: a review of patient and clinician variables. Canadian Journal of Psychiatry, 44(7), 665-670.

Kaplan, H. I., & Sadock, B. J. (2015). Kaplan and Sadock's Synopsis of Psychiatry. Philadelphia, PA: Wolters Kluwer.

Katterman, S. N., Kleinman, B. M., Hood, M. M., Nackers, L. M., & Corsica, J. A. (2014). Mindfulness meditation as an intervention for binge eating, emotional eating, and weight loss: A systematic review. Eating Behaviors, 15(2), 197-204.

Katzman, D. K., Peebles, R., Sawyer, S. M., Lock, J., & Le Grange, D. (2013). The role of the pediatrician in family-based treatment for adolescent eating disorders: Opportunities and challenges. Journal of Adolescent Health, 53(4), 433-440.

Kaye, W. H., Bulik, C. M., Thornton, L., Barbarich, N., & Masters, K. (2009). Comorbidity of anxiety disorders with anorexia and bulimia nervosa. The American Journal of Psychiatry, 161(12), 2215-2221.

Kaye, W. H., Fudge, J. L., & Paulus, M. (2009). New insights into symptoms and neurocircuit function of anorexia nervosa. Nature Reviews Neuroscience, 10(8), 573-584.

Keel, P. K., & Klump, K. L. (2003). Are eating disorders culture-bound syndromes? Implications for conceptualizing their etiology. Psychological Bulletin, 129(5), 747-769.

Knight, S., Allen, J., & Melson, T. (2020). Personalized Nutrition Approaches in the Treatment of Eating Disorders. Journal of Personalized Medicine, 11(1), 1-17.

Le Grange, D., & Eisler, I. (2009). Family interventions in adolescent anorexia nervosa. Child and Adolescent Psychiatric Clinics of North America, 18(1), 159-173.

Le Grange, D., Hughes, E. K., Court, A., Yeo, M., Crosby, R. D., & Sawyer, S. M. (2019). Randomized clinical trial of parent-focused treatment and family-based treatment for adolescent anorexia nervosa.

Journal of the American Academy of Child & Adolescent Psychiatry, 58(8), 787-796.

Leichner, P., Steiger, H., Puentes-Neuman, G., & Perreault, M. (2003). Implications for psychiatrists of intrafamilial disagreement on the subject of food and weight. Comprehensive Psychiatry, 44(6), 483-487.

Levine, M. P., & Piran, N. (2019). Reflections on the role of prevention in the history of eating disorder research and practice: The past, the present, and the future. International Journal of Eating Disorders, 52(5), 538-549.

Levine, M. P., & Piran, N. (2019). Reflections on the role of prevention in the linkage between body dissatisfaction and eating disorders. Eating Behaviors, 34, 101299.

Lock, J., Couturier, J., & Agras, W. S. (2001). Comparison of long-term outcomes in adolescents with anorexia nervosa treated with family therapy. Journal of the American Academy of Child & Adolescent Psychiatry, 40(6), 686-693.

Lock, J., Le Grange, D., Agras, W. S., & Dare, C. (2001). Treatment Manual for Anorexia Nervosa: A Family-Based Approach. New York: Guilford Press.

Lock, J., Le Grange, D., Agras, W. S., & Dare, C. (2010). Treatment manual for anorexia nervosa: A family-based approach. Guilford Press.

Lock, J., Le Grange, D., Agras, W. S., Moye, A., Bryson, S. W., & Jo, B. (2010). Randomized clinical trial comparing family-based treatment with adolescent-focused individual therapy for adolescents with anorexia nervosa. Archives of General Psychiatry, 67(10), 1025-1032.

Miller, S. M., Guttman, S. A., & Chaitoff, A. (2021). The road to recovery: A pilot study of the effects of meal timing on the treatment of anorexia nervosa. The Journal of Treatment & Prevention, 29(2), 543-556.

National Alliance on Mental Illness. (2020). Taking care of yourself. Retrieved from https://www.nami.org/Support-Education/ Publications-Reports/Guide-to-Navigating-Mental-Health/Dealing-with-a-Loved-One's-Mental-Health-Condition/Taking-Care-of-Yourself

National Institute of Mental Health. (2018). Eating Disorders: About More Than Food. U.S. Department of Health and Human Services, National Institutes of Health.

Pearlman, A. T., Schvey, N. A., Gray, J. N., & Tanofsky-Kraff, M. (2017). Weight bias internalization and health: A systematic review. Obesity Reviews, 18(7), 782-794.

Perloff, R. M. (2014). Social media effects on young women's body image concerns: Theoretical perspectives and an agenda for research. Sex Roles, 71(11-12), 363-377.

Phillips, K. A., Wilhelm, S., Koran, L. M., Didie, E. R., Fallon, B. A., Feusner, J., & Stein, D. J. (2005). Body dysmorphic disorder: Some key issues for DSM-V. Depression and Anxiety, 14-18.

Pike, K. M., Walsh, B. T., Vitousek, K., Wilson, G. T., & Bauer, J. (2003). Cognitive behavior therapy in the posthospitalization treatment of anorexia nervosa. American Journal of Psychiatry, 160(11), 2046-2049.

Ramjan, L. M. (2004). Nurses and the 'therapeutic relationship': Caring for adolescents with anorexia nervosa. Journal of Advanced Nursing, 45(5), 495–503.

Smith, A. R., & Cook-Cottone, C. (2013). A review of family therapy as an effective intervention for anorexia nervosa in adolescents. Journal of Clinical Psychology in Medical Settings, 20(4), 425-438.

Smith, A. R., & Cook-Cottone, C. (2020). A review of family therapy as an effective intervention for anorexia nervosa in adolescents. Journal of Clinical Psychology, 76(1), 219-241.

Smith, A. R., Joiner, T. E., & Dodd, D. R. (2006). Cognitive specificity in internalizing and externalizing problems: A meta-analysis of Beck's content specificity hypothesis. Journal of Abnormal Psychology, 115(3), 472-484.

Smith, R., Thomsen, T., & Markward, N. (2020). Behavioral indicators of eating disorders: Observations and interventions. Clinical Psychology Review, 78, 123-134.

Steinberg, L., & Morris, A. S. (2001). Adolescent development. Annual Review of Psychology, 52, 83-110.

Steinglass, J. E., Sysko, R., Mayer, L., Berner, L. A., Schebendach, J., Wang, Y., ... & Walsh, B. T. (2011). Pre-meal anxiety and food intake in anorexia nervosa. Appetite, 57(3), 668-671.

Stice, E., & Whitenton, K. (2002). Risk factors for body dissatisfaction in adolescent girls: A longitudinal investigation. Developmental Psychology, 38(5), 669-678.

Thompson, J. K., & Stice, E. (2001). Thin-ideal internalization: Mounting evidence for a new risk factor for body-image disturbance and eating pathology. Current Directions in Psychological Science, 10(5), 181–183.

Thompson, R. A., & Sherman, R. T. (2010). Eating Disorders in Sport. Routledge.

Tiggemann, M. (2003). Media exposure, body dissatisfaction and disordered eating: Television and magazines are not the same. European Eating Disorders Review, 11(5), 418-430.

Tiggemann, M., & Slater, A. (2014). NetGirls: The Internet, Facebook, and body image concern in adolescent girls. International Journal of Eating Disorders, 47(6), 630-643.

Treasure, J., & Schmidt, U. (2001). Ready, willing, and able to change: Motivational aspects of the assessment and treatment of eating disorders. European Eating Disorders Review, 9(1), 4-23.

Treasure, J., Duarte, T. A., & Schmidt, U. (2020). Eating disorders. The Lancet, 395(10227), 899-911.

Treasure, J., Schmidt, U., & van Furth, E. (2015). Handbook of eating disorders (2nd ed.). John Wiley & Sons.

Treasure, J., Todd, G., & Brolly, M. (2005). Why does anorexia still not get better in the 21st century? Therapeutic engagement in anorexia nervosa. European Eating Disorders Review, 13(6), 421-430.

Vitousek, K., Watson, S., & Wilson, G. T. (1998). Enhancing motivation for change in treatment-resistant eating disorders. Clinical Psychology Review, 18(4), 391-420.

Wang, G. J., Geliebter, A., Volkow, N. D., Telang, F. W., Logan, J., Jayne, M. C., ... & Fowler, J. S. (2011). Enhanced striatal dopamine release during food stimulation in binge eating disorder. Obesity, 19(8), 1601-1608.